The Ultimate Guide To Workouts And Kegel Exercises

A Step-By-Step Kegel Exercise Guide And Tips For 2x Strength Gains & Achieving Bodybuilding Goals With An Ultimate Diet Plan

Michael Kessler

Table of Contents

CHAPTER ONE 4
    Kegel Exercises 4
    The Purpose and Benefits of Kegel Exercises 5
    People That Benefit from Kegel Exercises 8
    Methods used in kegel exercise 10

CHAPTER TWO 15
    Effective Techniques for Kegel Exercises 15
    Kegel Exercises during Pregnancy 17
    Performing Kegel Exercises 19
    Locating Pelvic Floor Muscles 21
    Strengthening Pelvic Floor Muscles 22
    Step-by-Step Guide to Perform Kegel Exercises 23

CHAPTER THREE 26
    Identifying Correct Kegel Exercise Techniques 26
    Optimizing Kegel Exercises 27
    Pressure and Duration for Successful Kegels 29
    Additional Tips for Optimizing Kegel Exercises 31
    Ideal Positions for Kegel Exercises 33

CHAPTER FOUR 36
    Challenges and Solutions 36
    Common Issues with Kegel Exercises 37
    Benefits of Kegel Balls 39
    Results and Timelines 40
    Men Benefit from Kegel Exercises 42
    Conclusion 43

THE END..47

CHAPTER ONE

Kegel Exercises

Kegel exercises are a set of exercises designed to strengthen the pelvic floor muscles. These muscles support the bladder, uterus, and bowel. The exercises involve contracting and relaxing the pelvic floor muscles, which can help improve urinary incontinence, support recovery after childbirth, and enhance sexual function by increasing awareness and control of these muscles. They're often recommended for both men and women to maintain pelvic floor health.

The Purpose and Benefits of Kegel Exercises

Kegel exercises involve the repetitive contraction and relaxation of the pelvic floor muscles. The primary purpose is to strengthen these muscles, which support the bladder, uterus, small intestine, and rectum. Here's why they're beneficial:

Improving Bladder Control: Strengthening the pelvic floor muscles can help prevent or alleviate urinary incontinence, both in men and women. It can be especially helpful for stress incontinence, where there's leakage due to physical activity, sneezing, or laughing.

Enhancing Sexual Function: Stronger pelvic floor muscles can lead to increased sexual satisfaction for both partners. They can help with achieving and maintaining erections in men and improving vaginal tone and sensation in women.

Aiding in Postpartum Recovery: Pregnancy and childbirth can weaken pelvic floor muscles. Doing Kegel exercises postpartum can aid in faster recovery and help prevent issues like urinary incontinence.

Supporting Pelvic Organs: A strong pelvic floor provides support for pelvic organs, reducing the risk of pelvic organ prolapse, where organs like the bladder, uterus, or rectum can drop into the vaginal area.

Improving Bowel Function: Strengthening these muscles can also help with bowel control and prevent fecal incontinence.

Kegel exercises are relatively easy to do, and when performed consistently, they can have significant benefits for pelvic health. However, it's crucial to learn the correct technique and frequency to maximize their effectiveness.

People That Benefit from Kegel Exercises

Methods of Kegel Exercises Different Types of Kegel Exercises

Kegel exercises can benefit various groups of people:

Women:

- **During Pregnancy:** Helps prepare for childbirth and aids in postpartum recovery.

- **Postpartum:** Assists in restoring pelvic floor strength after childbirth.

- **In General:** Helps with bladder control, especially for those experiencing stress incontinence or urinary leakage.

Men:

- **Erectile Dysfunction:** Can assist in improving erectile function by enhancing blood flow and strengthening pelvic floor muscles.

- **Urinary Incontinence:** Helpful for men dealing with urinary leakage post-surgery, such as prostate surgery.

Seniors:

- Helps with age-related weakening of pelvic muscles, reducing the risk of urinary and fecal incontinence.

Methods used in kegel exercise

Kegel exercises can be done using different methods:

Regular Contractions: The standard method involves squeezing the pelvic floor muscles for a few seconds and then relaxing them for the same duration.

Quick Contractions (Flutter Kegels): Rapidly contract and relax the pelvic floor muscles, as if you're quickly stopping and starting urination.

Elevator Kegels: Gradually contract the pelvic floor muscles in a gentle upward "elevator" motion, increasing the intensity as if you're moving up floors in an elevator. Then slowly release them in reverse order.

Resistance Training: Some devices and tools offer resistance against which the pelvic floor muscles can contract, providing additional strength training.

Biofeedback and Electrical Stimulation: These methods involve using specialized devices that provide feedback or electrical stimulation to help identify and strengthen pelvic floor muscles.

Slow Contractions: Gradually contracting the pelvic floor muscles and holding the contraction for a few seconds (usually 5 to 10 seconds) before slowly releasing them.

Integrated Exercises: Incorporating pelvic floor exercises into other workouts like yoga, Pilates, or core exercises, integrating these muscles into a broader routine.

Electrical Stimulation: Some devices use electrical impulses to stimulate the pelvic floor muscles, helping to activate and strengthen them.

Relaxation Techniques: Learning to relax and release tension in the pelvic floor muscles is also essential. This prevents overexertion and maintains healthy muscle tone.

CHAPTER TWO
Effective Techniques for Kegel Exercises

- To ensure you're engaging the correct muscles, try to stop the flow of urine midstream once to identify the pelvic floor muscles. However, don't make a habit of doing Kegels while urinating, as it might disrupt bladder function.

- Sit, stand, or lie down comfortably. Focus on isolating the pelvic floor muscles without tensing your abdomen, thighs, or buttocks.

- Start with slow, gentle contractions, holding the squeeze for a few seconds before releasing. Gradually increase the duration of contractions as you build strength.
- Ensure to completely relax the muscles between contractions. Relaxation is as important as the contraction itself.
- Aim for consistency in practicing Kegel exercises. Start with a few sets of repetitions each day and gradually increase both the repetitions and the hold duration.

Kegel Exercises during Pregnancy

Preparation for Birth: Kegel exercises during pregnancy can help prepare the pelvic floor muscles for childbirth. Regular practice may aid in labor and postpartum recovery.

Bladder Control: Pregnant individuals often experience increased pressure on the bladder. Strengthening the pelvic floor muscles through Kegel exercises can assist in controlling urinary leakage or incontinence.

Consultation: It's crucial to consult with a healthcare professional before starting or continuing any exercise regimen during pregnancy. They can provide personalized guidance and ensure the exercises are safe for your specific situation.

Comfortable Positions: Experiment with different positions (sitting, standing, lying down) to find the most comfortable and effective way to perform Kegels during pregnancy.

Pacing and Caution: Avoid overexertion. While exercising the pelvic floor muscles is beneficial, excessive strain or fatigue might be counterproductive.

Performing Kegel Exercises

Regular Routine: Make Kegel exercises a part of your daily routine. Consider associating them with specific daily activities to help remember to do them consistently.

Monitoring Progress: Keep track of your progress. Notice any changes in bladder control or muscle strength over time.

Posture and Breathing: Maintain good posture and normal breathing while performing Kegel exercises. Avoid holding your breath or tensing other muscles.

Professional Guidance: If needed, seek guidance from a pelvic floor physical therapist or healthcare professional, especially if you're unsure about the correct technique or experiencing any discomfort.

Remember, Kegel exercises are generally safe for most people, but it's essential to perform them correctly and seek guidance if you have any concerns, especially during pregnancy.

Locating Pelvic Floor Muscles

- To identify the pelvic floor muscles, try stopping the flow of urine while using the restroom. However, don't make a habit of doing Kegels during urination, as it can lead to bladder issues.

- Another way to locate these muscles is by imagining stopping passing gas by contracting the muscles around the anus.

Strengthening Pelvic Floor Muscles

- Sit, stand, or lie down comfortably. Relax your abdomen, thighs, and buttocks.

- Contract the pelvic floor muscles without tensing other nearby muscles. Squeeze as if trying to stop urine flow without holding your breath.

- Hold the contraction for a few seconds, aiming for 5 seconds initially, then gradually increase the hold duration up to 10 seconds.

Release and relax for an equal amount of time.

- Perform sets of repetitions, starting with 10 repetitions per set. Gradually increase the number of repetitions as your muscles strengthen.

Step-by-Step Guide to Perform Kegel Exercises

Find a Comfortable Position: Sit, stand, or lie down comfortably, ensuring you're relaxed and can focus on isolating the pelvic floor muscles.

Identify Pelvic Floor Muscles: Use the methods mentioned earlier to locate the muscles you'll be engaging.

Contract and Hold: Squeeze the pelvic floor muscles as instructed, holding the contraction for the desired duration (start with 5 seconds).

Relaxation Phase: Release and relax the muscles for the same duration as the contraction.

Repeat and Gradually Increase: Perform sets of repetitions, gradually increasing both the hold duration and the number of repetitions as your muscles become stronger.

CHAPTER THREE
Identifying Correct Kegel Exercise Techniques

- Ensure you're isolating the pelvic floor muscles without involving nearby muscle groups like the abdomen, thighs, or buttocks.

- Avoid excessive force. The contractions should be gentle yet firm.

- Maintain normal breathing throughout the exercises. Avoid holding your breath, as this can cause unnecessary tension.

- Consistency is key. Make Kegel exercises a routine part of your day for optimal results.
- If unsure, consider consulting a pelvic floor physical therapist or healthcare professional for guidance on correct technique and personalized exercises.

Optimizing Kegel Exercises

Optimizing Kegel exercises involves assessing pelvic floor strength and understanding key factors like pressure and duration for successful exercises:

Assessing Pelvic Floor Strength:

Self-Assessment: Pay attention to improvements in bladder control, reduced instances of urinary leakage, or increased sensation in the pelvic region. These improvements can indicate enhanced pelvic floor strength.

Consultation: Consider consulting a pelvic floor physical therapist or healthcare professional for a more accurate assessment. They can use specialized techniques to evaluate pelvic floor strength and recommend tailored exercises.

Pressure and Duration for Successful Kegels

Pressure Control: Focus on applying just enough pressure to engage the pelvic floor muscles without straining or overexerting them. It's crucial to avoid excessive force, as this can lead to muscle fatigue or discomfort.

Gradual Progression: Start with a moderate level of pressure during contractions, gradually increasing as your muscles strengthen. Avoid sudden or drastic increases in pressure, as this might cause strain.

Duration of Contractions: Begin with shorter hold durations (around 5 seconds) during contractions and gradually extend the hold time as your muscles become stronger. Aim to reach a comfortable duration, typically around 10 seconds, without causing discomfort.

Relaxation Period: Equally important to contraction is the relaxation phase. Ensure you release the muscles fully and allow them to relax for the same duration as the contraction.

Additional Tips for Optimizing Kegel Exercises

Consistency: Establish a regular routine for Kegel exercises. Daily practice, with gradual increases in pressure and duration, leads to more effective strengthening of the pelvic floor muscles.

Quality over Quantity: Focus on the quality of contractions rather than the quantity. Proper technique and engagement of the correct muscles are crucial for effectiveness.

Variation and Progression: Introduce variations in your exercises, such as different types of contractions or incorporating resistance training tools. Progress gradually and listen to your body's response.

Professional Guidance: If in doubt or experiencing discomfort, seek guidance from a healthcare professional. They can offer personalized advice, correct technique, and exercises tailored to your needs.

Optimizing Kegel exercises involves a balanced approach, gradually increasing pressure and duration while maintaining proper technique and regular practice.

Pay attention to your body's signals and adjust the exercises accordingly to achieve optimal pelvic floor strength.

Ideal Positions for Kegel Exercises

The choice between sitting and standing positions for Kegel exercises often depends on personal comfort and effectiveness. Both positions offer benefits and challenges:

Sitting Position:

Comfort: Sitting may be more comfortable for many individuals, providing stability and a relaxed posture.

Convenience: It's easier to focus on isolating the pelvic floor muscles while seated, especially when starting Kegel exercises.

Ease of Practice: Doing Kegels while sitting can easily be integrated into daily activities, such as while working at a desk or watching TV.

Standing Position:

Functional Engagement: Standing engages the pelvic floor muscles differently, mimicking real-life scenarios where these muscles are often active (e.g., walking, standing).

Variation: Changing positions while exercising the pelvic floor can provide a more comprehensive workout for these muscles.

Challenge: Standing might present challenges in isolating the pelvic floor muscles for beginners.

CHAPTER FOUR

Challenges and Solutions

Isolation Difficulty: Some individuals find it challenging to isolate the pelvic floor muscles, especially when standing. Solution: Start practicing Kegels in a seated position initially to master muscle isolation before progressing to standing exercises.

Engagement Issues: Maintaining consistent engagement of the pelvic floor muscles throughout the exercise can be difficult. Solution: Focus on regular practice to improve muscle control and ensure you're not overexerting or holding your breath.

Difficulty Maintaining Posture: Maintaining proper posture while standing might be a challenge. Solution: Practice against a wall or use a stable surface for support until you gain better control of the muscles.

Common Issues with Kegel Exercises

Lack of Progress: If you're not experiencing improvements, reassess your technique. Ensure you're engaging the correct muscles and gradually increasing pressure and duration over time.

Discomfort or Pain: If you're experiencing discomfort or pain during or after Kegel exercises, consult a healthcare professional. They can evaluate your technique and suggest modifications or alternative exercises.

Inconsistent Practice: Staying consistent with Kegel exercises is crucial. Create reminders or associate the exercises with daily activities to maintain a regular routine.

Benefits of Kegel Balls

Kegel balls, also known as Ben Wa balls, are small, weighted devices designed to help with Kegel exercises by adding resistance and providing feedback. They are inserted into the vagina and are held in place by the pelvic floor muscles.

Strengthens Pelvic Floor: The added weight of Kegel balls challenges the pelvic floor muscles, enhancing their strength and control.

Improved Sensation: Some users report increased vaginal tone and enhanced sexual sensation after using Kegel balls regularly.

Bladder Control: Strengthening the pelvic floor can aid in better bladder control, reducing instances of urinary leakage or incontinence.

Results and Timelines

The timeline for noticing changes with Kegel exercises, including those involving Kegel balls, varies among individuals. Factors like consistency, effort, and initial muscle strength influence the timeline.

Short-Term Changes: Some individuals may notice improvements in muscle awareness and control within a few weeks of consistent practice.

Medium-Term Changes: Enhanced bladder control and reduced instances of urinary leakage might become noticeable within a few months of regular exercise.

Long-Term Changes: Significant improvements in pelvic floor strength and potential sexual benefits might become more apparent after several months of dedicated practice.

Men Benefit from Kegel Exercises

Men can benefit from Kegel exercises in various ways:

Improved Bladder Control: Kegel exercises can aid in reducing urinary incontinence, particularly after prostate surgery.

Enhanced Sexual Function: Strengthening the pelvic floor muscles can assist in improving erectile function and ejaculation control.

Pelvic Health: Building stronger pelvic floor muscles can contribute to better overall pelvic health and stability.

Men can perform Kegel exercises using similar techniques as women, by identifying and isolating the pelvic floor muscles and performing contractions and relaxations. Consistency and proper technique are key for men to experience the benefits of Kegel exercises.

Conclusion

Kegel exercises are valuable for strengthening the pelvic floor muscles, benefiting both men and women. These exercises, whether done conventionally or with aids like Kegel balls, offer numerous advantages:

Pelvic Floor Strength: They improve pelvic floor muscle tone, aiding in better bladder control, reducing urinary incontinence, and preventing pelvic organ prolapse.

Enhanced Sexual Function: Strengthening these muscles can contribute to improved sexual satisfaction, increased vaginal tone, and better erectile function.

Postpartum Recovery: Kegel exercises can aid in postpartum recovery by restoring pelvic floor strength and helping with any issues related to childbirth.

Individualized Benefits: The benefits and timelines for noticing changes vary among individuals and depend on consistency, effort, and initial muscle strength.

Whether done in sitting or standing positions, with Kegel balls or through conventional exercises, the key lies in consistent practice, proper technique, and gradually increasing pressure and duration.

THE END

www.ingramcontent.com/pod-product-compliance
Lightning Source LLC
Chambersburg PA
CBHW072020230526
45479CB00008B/310